THE LITTLE BOOK OF
MINDFULNESS

JENNIFER CORDERO

An Hachette UK Company
www.hachette.co.uk

Vie Books, an imprint of Summersdale Publishers
Part of Octopus Publishing Group Limited
Carmelite House
50 Victoria Embankment
LONDON
EC4Y 0DZ
UK

This FSC® label means that materials and other controlled sources used for the product have been responsibly sourced

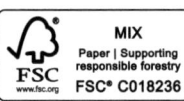

MIX
Paper | Supporting
responsible forestry
FSC® C018236

www.summersdale.com

The authorized representative in the EEA is Hachette Ireland, 8 Castlecourt Centre, Dublin 15, D15 XTP3, Ireland (email: info@hbgi.ie)

Printed and bound in the Poland

ISBN: 978-1-83799-624-7
eISBN: 978-1-83799-625-4

Substantial discounts on bulk quantities of Summersdale books are available to corporations, professional associations and other organizations. For details contact general enquiries: telephone: +44 (0) 1243 771107 or email: enquiries@summersdale.com.

Neither the author nor the publisher can be held responsible for any injury, loss or claim – be it health, financial or otherwise – arising out of the use, or misuse, of the suggestions made herein. This book is not intended as a substitute for the medical advice of a doctor or physician. If you are experiencing problems with your physical or mental health, it is always best to follow the advice of a medical professional.

CONTENTS

✦ INTRODUCTION ✦

Welcome to *The Little Book of Mindfulness*, a gentle guide that invites you to explore the transformative power of mindfulness. The pace of life in today's modern world can often leave us feeling emotionally overwhelmed and physically depleted. Mindfulness has emerged as an accessible path to cultivating greater physical, mental and emotional well-being. This ancient yet timeless approach to life encourages us to pause, breathe and connect, offering refuge from the stressors of modern life.

In this book, you'll learn more about the origins of mindfulness and how it has evolved into its contemporary model. You'll also be introduced to simple and practical mindfulness techniques that can

be seamlessly integrated into your daily life. Whether you're entirely new to mindfulness or wish to deepen your practice, you'll find a range of exercises designed to help you live more fully in the present moment. From mindful meditation to mindfulness in nature, you'll discover ways to reduce stress, increase self-awareness and improve your overall well-being.

As you dive in, you will find inspiration and calm within these pages. May this book be your trusted companion on your journey to a more mindful and balanced life.

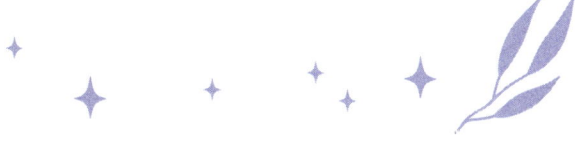

CHAPTER ONE

MINDFULNESS
101

In this chapter, you'll explore the concept of mindfulness – what it is, how it differs from meditation, its historical roots and its many benefits. Though often grouped together, mindfulness and meditation have some very different characteristics. You'll learn about the development of mindfulness, from its ancient beginnings to its modern applications in mental health and wellness. You'll also discover how mindfulness can positively affect physical and psychological well-being with its ability to reduce stress, improve emotional resilience and enhance focus, making it an essential tool for navigating today's fast-paced world.

✦ WHAT IS MINDFULNESS? ✦

Mindfulness is the art of paying and holding attention to the present moment, accepting all that comes without judgement. Paying attention is being aware of everything happening in and around you in the present moment. Holding attention means staying present throughout the experience of your thoughts and feelings without becoming overly involved.

Modern-day mindfulness has no end goal. It's not a way to stop thoughts. It's simply about becoming aware when your mind wanders to the past or future and continuously drawing it back to the present. While engaging in this "present moment awareness", mindfulness encourages you to resist becoming overwhelmed by any thoughts, feelings or emotions that arise.

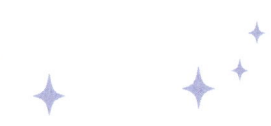

Mindfulness versus meditation

Although meditation can lead to a state of mindfulness, they are not the same thing. Many people find mindfulness more accessible as a concept and attainable as a practice. In meditation, the goal is to quieten the mind. Mindfulness is more about attention and awareness, concepts we all instinctively understand and, to some degree, already practise daily.

A main differentiation between meditation and mindfulness that can be hard to wrap our heads around is that mindfulness isn't temporary or situational. It's not something we practise at a specific time and then stop. Mindfulness is a way of moving through life, while meditation is more of a specific act that can help us to be more mindful.

Mindfulness is a skill (or an art!) that can grow and take on momentum in our lives so that it becomes almost automatic and habitual to live more mindfully. Think of meditation as going to the gym and exercising to build your muscles, while mindfulness is the muscle memory that grows stronger with each training session and that helps you to move through life more efficiently.

✦ MINDFULNESS ✦ IN MODERN LIFE

With so many external stimuli competing for our attention these days, it's easy to become overwhelmed by the constant hum of life. In addition to outside input, our internal dialogue can be off and running at a hare's pace without us even being aware. It's like standing in the middle of a powerful waterfall, with thoughts and feelings rushing toward and all around you. If you stay in the middle of that mighty deluge, you remain reactive to those thoughts. By stepping outside the flow, you can watch the waterfall without becoming a part of it.

Another benefit of practising mindfulness is that our pace of life seems to slow down. When we are more aware of each moment, our relationship to time changes, and we can deepen our appreciation for the rich fabric of life. Instead of feeling like our days and weeks are flashing by, developing our connection with the present moment will leave us feeling more fulfilled and satisfied.

A BRIEF HISTORY OF MINDFULNESS

The roots of mindfulness can be traced back to the Vedic period (*c.*1500–500 BCE). The earliest known reference of mindful self-awareness practices is from a collection of Vedic texts composed in the northern Indian subcontinent. These Vedic teachings were eventually incorporated into Hinduism. Later on, around 500 BCE, Siddhartha Gautama (the Buddha) developed his own teachings on mindful self-awareness.

The first known English translation of the concept dates from the 1880s when Thomas William Rhys Davids translated the Pali term *sati* into "mindfulness". The Buddhist concept of *sati* is widely understood to mean "moment-to-moment awareness of events", combined with "remembering to be aware of something".

Buddhist *Zazen* (or Zen meditation) is another practice that contributed to the development of mindfulness – but while *Zazen* remains rooted in Buddhism, with practitioners aiming for enlightenment, mindfulness is a secular practice that doesn't aim for a state of enlightenment.

THE HISTORY OF
WESTERN MINDFULNESS

In the 1960s, the concept of mindfulness migrated to the US via well-known Asian spiritualist teachers, including Zen teacher Thích Nhất Hạnh and Buddhist monk and scholar Nyanaponika Thera. Throughout the 1960s and 70s, many Americans travelled to Asia to learn about mindfulness.

One of Thích Nhất Hạnh's students, Jon Kabat-Zinn, went on to become a leading figure in the movement, bringing mindfulness to the Western world. Kabat-Zinn founded the Center for Mindfulness at the University of Massachusetts in the US and developed his eight-week Mindfulness-Based Stress Reduction (MBSR) course, a programme still widely used throughout the Western world today.

Other mindfulness pioneers in the West include Sharon Salzberg, Jack Kornfield, Joseph Goldstein and Jacqueline Schwartz Mandell, founders of the Insight Meditation Society (IMS) in Massachusetts. Salzberg, Kornfield and Goldstein remain high-profile figures in the mindfulness and meditation space.

✦ MINDFULNESS AND YOGA ✦

It's not a coincidence that in the West, interest in mindfulness has grown alongside the popularity of yoga. These two practices have long been intertwined, with the origins of yoga arising simultaneously as the development of Hinduism. Yet, like mindfulness, the westernized version of yoga has mainly de-emphasized the spiritual aspects of the practice to make it more attractive to the masses.

Most yoga disciplines stem from *The Yoga Sutras of Patanjali*, which outline the eight limbs (or elements) of yoga. The sutras offer guidance on how to live a life of purpose and meaning. The eight limbs include three mindful practices:

- **Dhāraṇā:** An intense concentration on one object to focus the mind in stillness.

- **Dhyāna:** Awareness without focus, judgement or attachment.

- **Pratyahara:** A removal of external distractions to enhance internal awareness.

MINDFULNESS IN OTHER TRADITIONS

Though mindfulness has clear origins in Hinduism and Buddhism, other spiritual and philosophical traditions include aspects of mindfulness.

Stoicism

In the third century BCE, Zeno founded Stoicism. Zeno shared the popular philosophy with his many disciples in Athens, including Roman statesman Seneca and Roman emperor Marcus Aurelius. At its heart, Stoicism is about being at peace throughout life's inevitable ups and downs. It includes mindfulness practices such as visualization exercises and nonjudgemental reactions.

Stoicism teaches that though we cannot control events, we can control how we react to them, thereby reducing the influence of external factors on our well-being. Centuries later, the Stoic concept of our thoughts affecting our emotions has formed part of modern-day cognitive behavioural therapy (CBT).

Christianity

Christian spiritual traditions also include some mindfulness concepts. In the sixteenth century, St Ignatius of Loyola penned a series of spiritual exercises, such as "Rules for Eating", which include mindful principles like focusing on what is being consumed and eating slowly.

Some Christians believe that prayer is a form of mindfulness; however, there's still strong resistance to mindfulness from others who view it as too intertwined with other religions. That said, Christianity has a long history of contemplative prayer, dating back to the third century, when it was practised by Christian hermits and monks living in the Egyptian desert. In the fourteenth century, *The Cloud of Unknowing*, written by an anonymous monk, suggested that humans could only access the divine through contemplative practices.

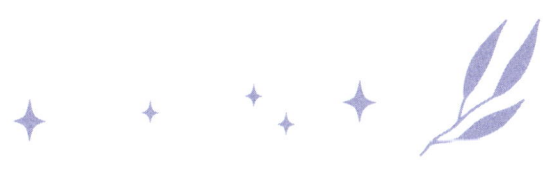

Transcendentalism

The philosophical and spiritual movement of transcendentalism originated in New England in the late 1820s when a handful of ministers, reformists and writers came together to form a club. The Transcendental Club included influential writers Ralph Waldo Emerson, Henry David Thoreau, Margaret Fuller and Henry Wadsworth Longfellow. Transcendentalism sprung from the understanding that "the mind had become aware of itself", which is similar to the mindfulness concept of watching one's thoughts.

Transcendentalism marked one of the first times in the West that groups began moving away from structured religions to more spiritual ways of thinking and living.

Teachings emphasized transcending the human experience through spiritual growth. Transcendentalist literature promoted immersion in nature and contemplation practices as ways to discover one's inner landscape. One of the movement's most famous founders, Henry David Thoreau, wrote about going to the woods to "live deliberately", poetically describing the very idea of mindfulness – that of present moment awareness.

Nowhere can man find a quieter or more untroubled retreat than in his own soul.

MARCUS AURELIUS

✦ MODERN-DAY MINDFULNESS ✦

In the late 1970s, there was a determined shift away from the connection between mindfulness and Buddhism in the US. The father of this movement is Jon Kabat-Zinn, who developed the Mindfulness-Based Stress Reduction (MBSR) programme. MBSR was introduced as an intervention to treat patients with chronic pain and later developed into a stress-management intervention tool.

A dedicated meditator, Kabat-Zinn admits to deliberately separating the fundamental principles of mindfulness meditation taught by the Buddha from Buddhism itself. His aim was to protect against the risk of MBSR being viewed as New Age, Eastern mysticism or religious and to allow the technique to be judged and appreciated for its scientific value.

The practices were so successful that the principles are now regularly taught to students undertaking medical degrees. In the 2000s, the MBSR principles were adapted to extend beyond medical settings and began to be used in schools, workplaces and prisons.

✦ MBSR ✦

The most widely known **MBSR** programme is an eight-week course that includes formal and informal mindfulness practices, including body scans, eating meditation and walking meditation.

The formal and informal practices, coupled with yoga, aim to enhance awareness of the transient nature of all thoughts, feelings and emotions.

Today, the **MBSR** programme is used in formal medical settings to help patients cope with physical symptoms of long-term illnesses, as well as to treat and relieve various other conditions including, but not limited to: anxiety, depression, stress, sleep problems, migraines, chronic pain, diabetes and cancer.

MBSR programmes are now taught by thousands of providers throughout the world both online and in person. There are also **MBSR**-based retreats (again, online and in person) run by reputable organizations.

POPULARIZATION AND CRITICISM

There's no doubt that mindfulness has become a mainstay in Western society. However, the secularization of fundamental practices rooted in Hinduism and Buddhism has not gone without criticism. By separating mindfulness from the ethical boundaries of religion and the end goal of enlightenment, does it just end up being a form of self-discipline disguised as self-help? In other words, does mindfulness simply teach us how to cope instead of helping with the original aim of liberation from attachment or a false sense of self?

An interesting distinction between mindfulness in the East and the West is how it is used and applied. In the East, mindfulness is seen by many as a daily practice and a routine way of life. In the West, mindfulness is viewed more as a treatment, a cure or an act that one does – e.g. attending a mindfulness class or studying mindfulness as a form of self-improvement.

Cultural appropriation

Modern-day mindfulness has come under scrutiny for its cultural whitewashing. By separating mindfulness from its roots and origins to satisfy Western ways of life, we risk losing its authenticity. While adapting the practices to be more universally accessible has value, it's equally important to give due recognition to its cultural roots and heritage.

McMindfulness

While one might argue that the secularization of mindfulness has made it accessible to more people, the downside is that it has also left mindfulness open to rampant commercialization and the use of mindfulness as a marketing tool. In 2011, Buddhist psychotherapist and meditation teacher Miles Neale coined the phrase "McMindfulness" to describe the current trend of meditation for the masses. He likened it to a mass-produced meal that might look, smell and taste good but is void of any nutrition and likely to quickly leave you feeling hungry again.

Heavily meditated

Mass commercialization of mindfulness is underway, with the mindfulness "industry" currently valued in the billions and set to grow. There are classes and courses to teach mindfulness, app-assisted mindfulness meditations and even tech-enabled meditation headbands that act as personal meditation coaches. While experts agree that the benefits of practising a secular style of mindfulness are plentiful, there remain downsides to separating the tradition from its origin.

Why origin matters

Recognizing the roots of mindfulness pays proper respect to its cultural heritage, avoiding the pitfalls of cultural appropriation and adding authenticity to the practice.

With mindfulness becoming a buzzword used to sell everything from T-shirts to tea, it's important to recognize that mindfulness is a powerful practice grounded in spirituality. Mindfulness is an act of quiet contemplation, so in many ways it's hard to see how adding wearable tech might enhance this. It's possible, and arguably preferable, to practise mindfulness without special clothing, cushions or high-tech headbands.

Mindfulness helps us get better at seeing the difference between what's happening and the stories we tell ourselves about what's happening.

SHARON SALZBERG

✦ PHYSICAL BENEFITS ✦

Studies suggest that the benefits of mindfulness are wide-ranging, including boosting cognitive function, lowering the risk of heart disease and relieving symptoms of anxiety and depression. Some of the physical benefits of practising mindfulness include:

- **Better sleep:** Stress and anxiety are often contributing factors to poor sleep patterns. Practising mindfulness can decrease stress, which can lead to better sleep and increased energy levels.

- **Chronic pain relief:** Studies have found that a regular mindfulness practice can help to reduce the frequency and severity of chronic migraines. People who have fibromyalgia have also found it to be an effective pain-relief treatment.

- **Better overall health:** Undoubtedly, stress has a detrimental effect on our physical and mental well-being. Studies have shown that when we practise mindfulness, our overall health gets a boost as we start to look after ourselves more generally.

- **Improved cognitive function:** Even short bursts of mindfulness can improve short-term memory in the longer term. Mindfulness can also help prevent cognitive decline as we age by slowing down the effects of neuroinflammation.

- **Lower blood pressure:** A 2019 study of people with hypertension confirmed that practising mindfulness could lower both systolic and diastolic blood pressure, meaning mindfulness may decrease the risk of hypertension, coronary heart disease and type-2 diabetes.

- **Positive neuroplasticity changes:** The brain strives constantly to become more effective. Neuroplasticity is the process of reorganizing the brain, rewiring connections to achieve improved outcomes. Mindfulness can influence this rewiring, sending messages to our brain that we are more effective when we're aware and observant.

- **Stronger immune system:** Mindfulness can increase your body's ability to deal with infection and inflammation. Studies have shown that mindfulness can bolster an antibody response to infection and promote healing.

NEUROSCIENCE OF MINDFULNESS

Practising mindfulness can change your brain. Multiple studies have shown that the brain's neuroplasticity allows it to rewire existing neural connections and form new ones as we move through life. This means that even fleeting thoughts and feelings can leave a lasting impression on the brain – imagine the impact continuous emotions might have.

Mindfulness practice can help the brain form positive neural structures, leading to greater levels of joy, peace and happiness.

Neuroscientist Sara Lazar studied the effects of meditation on the brains of regular practitioners in their 40s and 50s. She found that meditation may help slow down age-related thinning of the frontal cortex, the area of the brain that contributes to the formation and retention of memories. In the study, Lazar found that regular meditators had the same amount of grey matter, a type of tissue crucial for day-to-day functioning, in their 40s and 50s as non-meditators in their 20s and 30s.

In a follow-up study, non-meditators attended an eight-week Mindfulness-Based Stress Reduction (MBSR) course. Researchers found that after eight weeks, brain volume had increased in four regions, including the hippocampus and the temporoparietal junction. The hippocampus is the area of the brain responsible for regulating emotion and storing memories, and the temporoparietal junction is responsible for empathy and compassion.

In addition, the study found a decrease in the amygdala area of the brain, which is responsible for the "fight or flight" response. The smaller the amygdala becomes, the easier it is to regulate the stress response. The study also found that the physical decrease in size correlated with reported changes in the participants' stress levels.

These studies provide positive correlations between mindfulness practices like meditation and an increased ability to manage stress and regulate emotions.

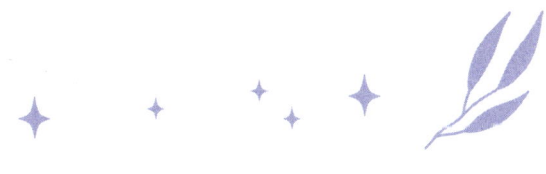

✦ MENTAL HEALTH BENEFITS ✦

Along with the neurological improvements that arise from practising mindfulness, some of the mental benefits practitioners report include:

- **Attitude of gratitude:** Tuning into the present moment leads to a greater appreciation of the beauty all around us. We start to appreciate simple joys, like the feeling of the sun on our faces or literally stopping to smell the flowers. Once we start appreciating our surroundings, the gratitude takes on its own momentum and increases our optimism. This helps us value what we have instead of fixating on any lack or shortcomings.

- **Decreased anxiety:** Mindfulness techniques that increase compassion and reduce tension can help manage anxiety and stress. Studies have shown regular mindfulness-based stress reduction practitioners report fewer worries and fears.

- **Fewer symptoms of depression:** Participation in mindfulness-based cognitive therapy can reduce the risk of relapse in people suffering from major depressive disorder. Mindfulness techniques that focus the mind on the present moment can help ease the effects of feeling mentally stuck, a concern that many people with depression report. Mindfulness can also help reduce the tendency to focus on problems rather than solutions.

- **Improved resilience:** Resilience is about managing stressful situations or circumstances and our ability to bounce back from adversity. Mindfulness can support both instances by giving us coping mechanisms to reduce stress and keep challenges in perspective when they arise.

- **Less reactiveness:** Learning to observe our thoughts and feelings makes us less likely to become one with them. This helps us become more measured in our responses rather than reactive. You're less likely to respond impulsively when you're aware of your emotions. Curbing impulsive behaviour makes more space for considered decision-making and, most likely, better outcomes.

- **Reduced cravings:** Research points to mindfulness helping to reduce addictive and compulsive behaviours. Mindfulness meditation decreases stress and improves overall mood, which can lead to fewer cravings. Similarly, mindful eating is associated with a lower risk of binge eating and can even support efforts to quit smoking. While mindfulness can't eliminate cravings, it can raise awareness of them, allowing for a choice of whether or not to indulge them.

- **Stress management:** The single most wide-reaching benefit of mindfulness is stress reduction, which has positive ripple effects both physically and mentally. When the mind is stressed, the body is stressed. Mindfulness can teach us to observe our stressors without reacting to them, which allows us to manage them more effectively.

Though there are many positive indications that mindfulness has both physical and mental benefits, its long-term effects are still relatively unstudied. The body of evidence will grow as mindfulness increases in popularity and general use in the West, but it is not a miracle cure or medical treatment.

LIMITATIONS IN MENTAL HEALTH MANAGEMENT

Despite having many wonderful benefits, mindfulness also has its limitations. Though only a small percentage of people experience an adverse effect from mindfulness, it's worth emphasizing that mindfulness is not a miracle cure.

Some reported negative side effects are disrupted sleep patterns, emotional blunting (becoming emotionless), societal withdrawal and feelings of reduced responsibility for one's actions. In some cases, increasing self-focused attention, such as body or breath awareness, can increase the intensity of emotions to the point of creating a stress response. Similarly, being able to observe your emotions can sometimes lead to feelings of disembodiment.

Finally, the mindfulness principle of staying present with one's emotions without engaging in them may prove troublesome for people who cannot move past certain emotions. For individuals who overly identify with feelings of guilt or fear, remaining present with those emotions might not be particularly helpful.

✦ COMMON MYTHS ✦
OF MINDFULNESS

Myth: Mindfulness is an ancient religion.
Truth: Though mindfulness developed alongside and within Buddhist and Hindu teachings, most current mindfulness practices are entirely secular.

Myth: Mindfulness is about emptying the mind.
Truth: Mindfulness is about becoming more aware of thoughts, emotions and feelings without becoming involved in them. There's no particular goal to stop thoughts from coming, though with practice, you might find you can break negative thought patterns.

Myth: Mindfulness is the same as relaxation.
Truth: While a mindfulness session might feel relaxing, it could also give rise to feelings of frustration, boredom or restlessness. By not engaging in the range of immediate emotions, we aim for a broader sense of contentment.

Myth: Mindfulness is only meditation.
Truth: Mindfulness can be practised through meditation, but it also can be practised in more informal ways, like mindful eating, walking and even

mindful spending. Engaging in a range of formal and informal techniques is a great way to turn mindfulness from something you do to something you are.

Myth: Mindfulness is a quick fix.
Truth: Beginners can often get discouraged at the start, wondering if "it's working". Instead of thinking of mindfulness as an easy and speedy solution, view it as an investment of time that can change your life for the better.

Myth: You need a quiet place to practise mindfulness.
Truth: Mindfulness can be practised anywhere at any time. While some formal mindfulness practices might benefit from a quiet space, many mindful opportunities arise throughout the day. We can be mindful when communicating, cooking and even while commuting!

Myth: Mindfulness will make you passive.
Truth: Sometimes, contentment is mistaken for a lack of conviction. However, we don't need to ride a rollercoaster of emotions to have strong goals and the determination to meet them. Mindfulness can help us reach our goals more easily by making us more resilient when faced with adversity.

✦ ADDRESSING SCEPTICISM ✦

We live in interesting times. Every day, we receive a barrage of information and stimulation from multiple directions. Most of us have personal devices that make us contactable 24 hours a day, seven days a week. We have deadlines to meet and dreams to chase. How on earth is sitting and staring into space going to help?

Here are some points of resistance that can arise when we first learn about mindfulness. Perhaps you'll encounter some of these same thoughts on your mindfulness journey!

I don't have time for mindfulness.
Mindfulness can help you prioritize your time, focus your attention and give you more energy – three things that will all make you more efficient throughout your day, leaving more time for mindfulness. That said, mindfulness doesn't have to take a long time to be effective. Informal mindfulness practices, like mindful cooking or eating, can be incorporated without taking you out of your day-to-day routines.

I'm too anxious to sit still and relax.

Saying this is rather like saying, "I'm too dirty to take a bath." That said, mindfulness doesn't require sitting still and relaxing. Mindfulness can be achieved by taking a walk outside in nature or going out for a jog, but instead of plugging in headphones, take the time to observe your surroundings as you go. Notice the sights, sounds and smells along your regular route, and you'll return home fitter in body and mind.

I'm not religious, and/or my religion prevents me from trying other spiritual practices.

Most modern-day mindfulness practices are neither religious nor spiritual. You don't have to be Buddhist, Hindu or even spiritually curious to enjoy the benefits of mindfulness.

It won't work quickly enough.

Mindfulness can have a powerful impact on our lives in a very short period, but it might take months before we notice any difference. That doesn't mean you're not reaping some of the benefits of mindfulness – they just might not be immediately apparent to you at the start of your journey. Still, mindfulness isn't a quick fix and shouldn't be considered one. Changing how you interact with your thoughts and emotions takes time and energy, but what you get in return is worth the effort.

I've tried it a few times; I'm not very good at it.

There's no one-size-fits-all when it comes to mindfulness. It can be practised in various settings and styles, with formal guidance or informal engagement. The beauty of this is that if you don't like counting your breaths or going to yoga, you can take a mindful walk at lunchtime or eat in a quiet place without trying to multi-task. But, like any new skill, learning mindfulness will take time, so don't get discouraged!

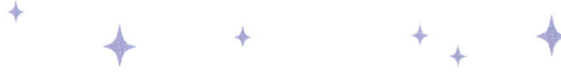

✦ SUMMARY ✦

Mindfulness is still relatively new to the West, and we're only just starting to see its potential (and learn about possible flaws) through formal scientific research. In the East, mindfulness is viewed by many as a way of life; it's also practised much more in the context of spirituality and community where it's rooted. The westernized version has become somewhat more individually focused. While both iterations can have pros and cons, knowing the framework from which mindfulness originated and evolved is important.

It's also helpful to remember that mindfulness is free. It doesn't cost anything to learn or practise and can be done in many different places. With its potential to address many modern-day ailments, mindfulness is marketed, monetized and packaged under sometimes hefty price tags. Certainly, classes and courses are available for those who prefer formal instruction or settings, but they are not the only ways to access mindfulness. If you're new to the practice, try a variety of techniques and you'll soon be building your mindfulness muscles in no time at all.

CHAPTER TWO

BASICS OF
MINDFULNESS

Mindfulness can be practised in many different ways. This chapter will explore the foundations of a mindfulness practice and look at various formal and informal practices. There are also some step-by-step exercises to get you started.

You might find some of the exercises easy and others more of a challenge. This is perfectly normal! The journey toward living more mindfully is an ever-evolving one and your practice will change as you gain experience and exposure. Though there are various mindfulness methods, they all share the same goal of cultivating calm and clarity while increasing awareness of thoughts and emotions.

✦ GETTING STARTED ✦

In the last chapter, we looked at the beneficial impact mindfulness can have on your life, but the list of positives doesn't end there. Mindfulness doesn't demand a great deal of preparation to get started. While it does require practice and patience, once you understand the fundamentals, you can drop moments of mindfulness into your daily routine.

Accessible to all

Mindfulness is free and can be used by anyone. It can be practised at any time and there's no need for any specialized equipment, clothing or a special place to practise (though you may find some environments more conducive and others more challenging to navigate – that's all part of the learning process).

Variety and versatility

There's no right or wrong way to practise mindfulness. You can choose to incorporate a range of exercises throughout different aspects of your life, or you can choose to focus on one area for improvement – perhaps being more mindful at work or in your relationships.

Personalizing your practice

We're all unique in our capacity for focusing attention, which is influenced by our life experiences, cultural influences and other factors. Understanding your strengths and weaknesses can help you tailor your mindfulness training to best accommodate these factors. Consider which you find hardest:

- Filtering distractions
- Holding something in awareness
- Managing the desire for stimulus

Ignoring these inherent aspects of yourself will lead to frustration and potentially giving up entirely. That's not to say that you should only ever work to your strengths – challenging a weakness is a great growth opportunity. Finding the balance between the two will help you navigate between achievement and improvement.

As you start exploring the different forms of formal and informal practices and dipping your toes into the exercises, remember that there is no single path to success. Becoming more mindful is a lifelong journey.

✦ THE THREE As OF MINDFULNESS ✦

The three As are core concepts of mindfulness that can help you develop a deeper connection with yourself, with others and with your environment. They are the foundation of any mindfulness practice.

Awareness
This is when you become alert to the thoughts, feelings, emotions and intentions that are present in your mind and body. Without awareness, many of these can go unnoticed, yet they can have a negative impact on us physically, mentally and emotionally. Recognizing their existence is the first step of any mindfulness journey.

Attention
Attention requires staying in the present moment as an observer. Once you notice thoughts and feelings arising, it's all too easy to let them take you down a path back in time or into the future. Paying attention, as we do when practising mindfulness, is not the same as focusing attention. There's no expectation that your mind will stay focused on one subject or object.

Acceptance

This means acknowledging where you are, how you got there and what is happening in the moment. This is perhaps the most challenging part of mindfulness: to accept the present situation as is, welcoming all experiences without judgement or shame.

Each of these actions requires us to take ownership of our thoughts, an important step in slowing down mindless mental chatter. When these three aspects of mindfulness are in play, we create a more spacious way of understanding and relating to ourselves and to others.

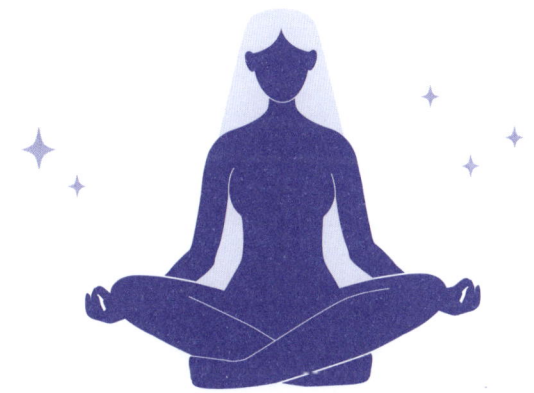

MINDFULNESS IN DIFFERENT CONTEXTS

One reason mindfulness is so accessible is its flexibility. Mindfulness can be practised in both formal and informal settings. It can be self-directed, you can study with a teacher or you can use apps to guide you through your session.

Informal mindfulness practices

There are many opportunities to add moments of mindfulness throughout your day. Informal mindfulness can bring surprising enjoyment to repetitive or routine tasks. Here are some ideas to get you started:

- **Begin with intention:** Set a clear intention at the start of your day, for example, "I will pause before speaking today." Return to the intention at set times throughout the day and reflect on how well you are sticking to the plan.

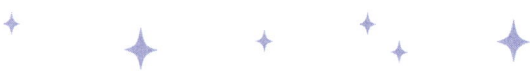

- **Communicate mindfully:** Mindful communication is a great way to make others feel heard and valued. In conversation with others, listen without planning your reply. Ask clarifying questions. Consider your choice of words and tone.

- **Eat mindfully:** Plan your mealtimes in advance and take time to sit and simply eat. Notice the texture of your food, how it looks, smells and tastes. Eat slowly. Savour each bite.

- **Listen to nothing:** Sound is a powerful stimulant. Music can soothe, and noise can agitate. We all have a soundtrack to our lives, whether it's through headphones or ambient, everyday sounds. Listening to nothing is simply taking in everything you can hear without judgement. Leave the headphones at home and see how many sounds you can identify throughout the day.

- **Walk mindfully:** When was the last time you really paid attention to where you were going when you were walking? Instead of popping your earbuds in the minute you hit the pavement, try walking without distraction. Even familiar routes will feel different when you take time to notice everything around you.

✦ OVERCOMING DISTRACTION ✦

Overcoming distraction is a skill that takes time to learn and years to master. Sometimes, it seems like our monkey minds wait until the very moment we're trying to focus our attention to start slinging arrows of distraction.

In truth, those thoughts likely exist under the surface anyway. We become aware of them when we start to become quiet. Training our minds to rest in attention is a continuous cycle of focus and distraction. The goal is to shorten the time between the mind wandering and becoming aware that it's happened.

In one mindfulness session, you'll likely complete this circular model many times, moving from fully focused to fully distracted and back again.

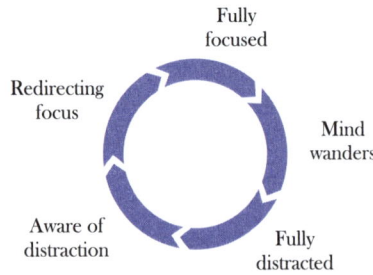

Fully focused

Redirecting focus

Mind wanders

Aware of distraction

Fully distracted

✦ MINDFULNESS MEDITATION: ✦ WHAT IS IT?

Mindfulness meditation is a powerful combination of the concept of mindfulness and the practice of meditation. Though mindfulness and meditation are interlinked, they are not synonymous. Where mindfulness is noticing thoughts, feelings and emotions as they arise, meditation trains the mind for focus and stillness to reach a state of calm. Together, mindfulness meditation is a practice of continuously drawing ourselves back to the present moment through focused attention.

Mindfulness meditation can be guided or self-directed. There's no minimum or maximum time limit on your practice. Even a few minutes a day, repeated over time, is a wonderful way to start building your attention and focus and can positively impact your overall well-being.

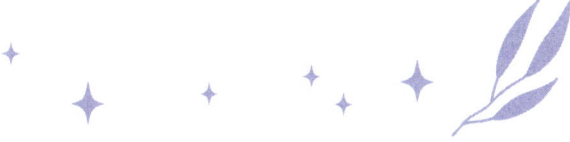

✦ GETTING STARTED ✦

Time

Choose a time of day that you can set aside for meditation. You may want to experiment with different times of day to see what works best, but consistency is key to creating a regular routine.

Duration

Set a timer for your practice. Try to resist the urge to keep looking to see how much time is left. Five minutes is an excellent starting length. You can build up in one-minute increments over time.

Space

Creating the right atmosphere for your meditation practice could help enhance the experience. A quiet place, free from distraction and interruption, is much more conducive to quiet contemplation than somewhere busy or used by others.

Practice

Remember that meditation is a practice. It takes time to learn and a lifetime to improve. There will be good days and bad days; it's not a linear process of progression to achieve a state of total calm and clarity. Try different ways of meditating, such as "watching the breath" and mantra meditation, which can be self-guided. There are also many apps and online resources for guided meditations.

Habit

Commitment is essential to learning, but what you'll get in return is well worth the time and effort. The most crucial moment of any single practice is the first one – showing up for yourself daily can have a profound effect.

Top tip: If you're new to formal meditation, start slowly and build up. It's better to practise for two minutes a day, five days a week, than to do only one ten-minute session weekly. Little and often is the best way to begin building your mindfulness meditation muscles.

EXERCISE: 5-4-3-2-1 GROUNDING

Engaging your five senses can help anchor you in the present. This is especially useful if your thoughts are drawn to the past or hurtling off into the future. To fully engage in your environment, try focusing your awareness on what you can see, hear, touch, smell and taste. To get started:

5 Name five things you can see in your immediate surroundings. Give some description to each one, noticing its size, shape and colour. Is there something you like about it or something you don't like?

4 Next, close your eyes and identify four sounds. Closing your eyes helps sharpen your hearing as you listen for noises close by, and then extend your hearing outward, listening for sounds in the distance. Note the pitch and volume of each. Are the sounds constant, or do they come and go?

3   Now move on to three things you can feel. This could be stroking a pet or noticing the fabric of your clothing. What is its texture? Does it feel hard? Soft? Smooth? What temperature is it?

2   Shift your awareness to your sense of smell, seeking out two distinct scents. If you're outside, can you smell flowers or rain? Inside, you might detect the aroma of brewing coffee or notice the fragrance of your clothing or hair products.

1   Finally, focus on one thing you can taste. If you're not eating or drinking at that moment, then try to recall your last meal or a favourite drink. Is it sweet or sour? Hot or cold? Crunchy or smooth?

Try engaging your senses to become fully aware of your environment and guide your thoughts firmly into the present.

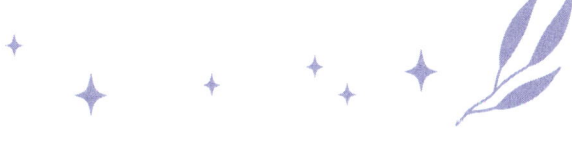

✦ EXERCISE: WISH ✦ YOU WERE HERE

Try this any time, but it's best to practise where there aren't too many distractions.

Start to think of a palm tree – maybe it's one you've seen in person, on a postcard or one you dream of sitting under on your next holiday. Begin examining the tree closely. What does the trunk look like? How tall is it? Where is it located? On the beach? In a garden? Keep building a detailed picture of that palm tree in your mind until you catch yourself thinking about something else entirely – perhaps what you'll have for lunch.

Now the fun begins. Trace your thoughts backward from what you're thinking about *(What's for lunch?)* to your palm tree. Try to remember each thought in the chain until you've returned to your tree. Practised regularly, you may notice that your path back to the palm tree gets shorter with time, which means you're becoming more aware of when your mind starts wandering.

BODY-SCAN MEDITATION: WHAT IS IT?

Body-scan meditation involves systematically moving through the physical body, noticing feelings and sensations without judgement. It's a beginner-friendly form of mindfulness that many people find relaxing. Body scans can be self-directed or guided. Apps and online resources are a great middle ground to help you get started.

Our physical bodies are often containers for our stress. Not only can we put physical strain on our bodies, but sometimes mental or emotional upset can manifest into physical blocks or tension. We can often ignore physical clues or flags, dismissing them as fleeting or temporary. Body-scan meditation is helpful for checking in and seeing what's happening without judgement.

Body scans are a fantastic way to reinforce the mind-body connection. Sometimes, we can get so caught up in our thoughts and emotions that we lose connection with our physical bodies. Living too much in our heads can lead to us feeling ungrounded and even manifest as clumsiness.

✦ GETTING STARTED ✦

Body-scan meditation is a form of mindfulness meditation. It can be done lying down; however, many people find that can lead to falling asleep, which is not the goal. Stay neutral when moving through the body, observing sensations without judgement.

Get comfortable

Settle into a comfortable position. Whether seated or lying down, you want to limit any adjusting or fidgeting, so take a few minutes to find the best position for you.

Close your eyes

Close your eyes or soften your gaze. Shutting the eyes is a great way to signal your intention to switch your awareness from looking outward to looking inward.

Begin with the breath

The breath is a gateway to the physical body. When beginning to practise a body-scan meditation, tuning into the breath serves as a form of grounding.

Start scanning

As you scan, begin to notice any sensations you are feeling in the body. What's happening that you may not have been attuned to?

Ease back to the present

You'll want to ease back into your surroundings gently. Take a few minutes to come back to the breath and then invite some gentle movement to the body, like wiggling the fingers and toes.

Top tip: When you feel agitated, notice any physical responses to the negative thoughts or feelings. Are you clenching your jaw? Hunching your shoulders? Understanding the link between the body and mental or emotional stress can help you turn the tide and begin to use physical relaxation to positively impact your thoughts and feelings.

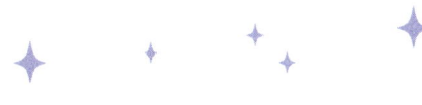

✦ EXERCISE: BODY SCAN ✦

Relax into a comfortable position. Soften your gaze, turning your awareness inward. Get ready to practise a short body scan.

1   Take a deep breath in and a full breath out. Bring your awareness to the top of your body: your head, face, neck and shoulders. Notice any sensations, movement or any areas where you might be holding on to tension or stress.

2   Move your awareness down to your arms, wrists and hands. Sense the back of the body and the front of the body. What feelings and sensations are present?

3   Bring your awareness to your lower body: legs, ankles and feet. Notice if there are any sensations or areas of tension.

4   Scan your entire body for sensations or movement. Turn your attention to your breath – notice the whole body breathing.

5   Finish your practice with a deep breath in and a full breath out.

There is nothing more important to true growth than realizing that you are not the voice of the mind — you are the one who hears it.

MICHAEL A. SINGER

YOGA ĀSANAS: WHAT ARE THEY?

Yoga āsanas are the physical presentation of yoga, alternatively known as yoga postures. Although they form only one part of a holistic yoga practice, the physical poses have become synonymous with most people's idea of yoga classes. Traditionally in Hatha and Ashtanga yoga (which form the basis of most yoga lineages today), āsanas were a way to prepare for meditation. They are a series of movements and breath work that originally aimed to quieten the body and mind so that it was possible to be still for long periods of meditation. Westernized versions of yoga may have traded philosophy for physicality, but yoga is still a popular way to practise mindfulness by keeping the focus on the body and breath.

Despite some images promoted in mainstream media, yoga is for everybody and *every* body. It's not reserved for the young and flexible, and you don't need to be able to touch your toes to reap the benefits of yoga. There are many different types and styles of yoga. Some are fast and physically demanding, some are slow but strong and others are gentle and incorporate lots of resting postures. There's even chair yoga, which doesn't require getting up and down from a yoga mat and can be great for people with restricted mobility.

> **Top tip:** Though it may seem that yoga studios are popping up everywhere, yoga is still very much a cottage industry. From big cities to rural villages, many independent teachers will hire spaces to set up their classes. Check local noticeboards or, for instance, church halls or community centres near you to see if there are any suitable classes.

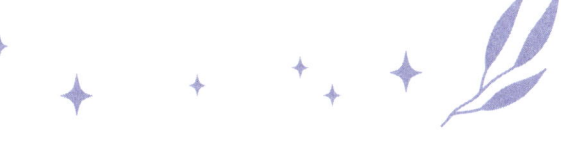

✦ GETTING STARTED ✦

Though you don't need yoga-specific clothing to get started, you will want to choose comfortable clothes you can easily move around in. Choose fuss-free options, avoiding anything too tight or excessively baggy. Try to minimize distractions; it might be helpful to tie up long hair and remove any jewellery. A yoga mat is a good idea as it helps you work on your alignment, offers extra padding and can help stop your hands and feet from slipping.

Yoga can be practised in many different settings. You might find a local beginner's class or there might be options at your local gym or leisure centre. There are many detailed books that you can learn from at your own pace. You can also explore online classes, many of which are accessible for free or for a small fee. Practising with a teacher can give you valuable feedback when you're just starting, but don't let that be a barrier to giving it a go if that's not possible. Keep in mind that everyone's body is different. You'll have to figure out what works for yours, and you'll want to always move in a way that feels good to you.

There are different ways to achieve a mindful yoga practice. For some, a strong and sweaty, physically challenging practice will be what they need to keep their mind focused. For others, incorporating a lot of pauses to check in with the breath or a continuous effort to coordinate breath and movement will create that connection. One series of postures that can help focus the mind are balancing postures – if you start thinking about what's for dinner while trying to stand on one leg in tree pose, you will soon find yourself falling out of that tree!

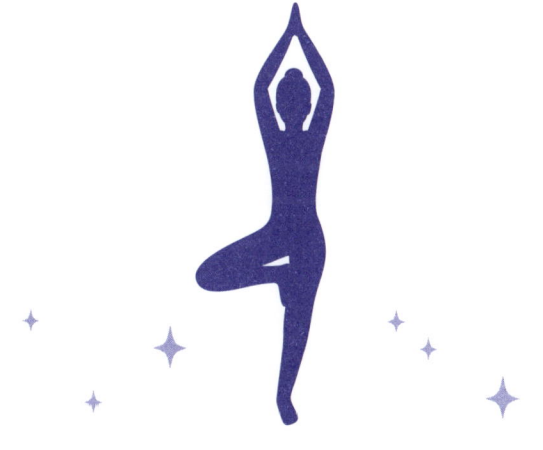

✦ EXERCISE: YOGA ĀSANAS ✦

Here are a few beginner-friendly yoga postures that bring together body and breath.

Child's Pose (*Bālāsana*)

Start on all fours, with your wrists under your shoulders and knees under your hips. Connect your big toes and spread your knees as wide as your yoga mat. Sink your belly in between your thighs as you extend your arms out in front of you. Rest your forehead on a block or rolled up towel if it doesn't touch the ground. Rest here for as long as you like. To release, place your hands underneath your shoulders and press back up to a tabletop position.

Top tip: Experiment with different positions for your arms – they can also rest by your side instead of extending forward.

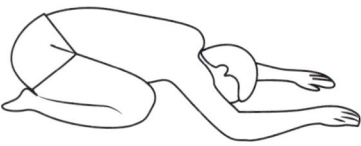

Mountain Pose (*Tāḍāsana*)

Come to standing with your feet hips-width apart. Lift your toes, spread them out and place them back onto the ground. Activate the muscles in your legs. Relax the shoulders and roll them forward, up and down, as if sliding your shoulder blades down the back. With arms resting by your sides, spread your fingers wide, palms facing forward. Keep your gaze steady, looking toward the horizon.

Top tip: If you find it hard to keep the legs active and engaged, try bending your knees slightly.

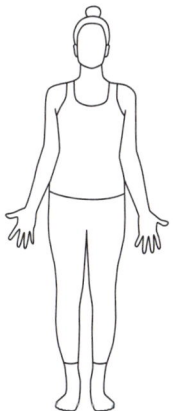

Tree Pose (Vrikshasana/*Vṛkṣāsana*)

From mountain pose, fix your gaze slightly higher than your regular line of sight. Shift your weight to your left leg and lift onto your right toes. Rotate your right knee outward, connecting the sole of the foot with the inside of the left ankle. Stay here or, if you like, lift the right foot higher to frame the calf of the left leg. If you're very flexible and stable, you can reach down for your right ankle and lift the foot above the left knee, so the sole of the foot is pressing against the inner left thigh.

Once steady, you can take your hands into a prayer position in front of your heart centre or lift them directly up to the sky. Hold for 30 seconds to one minute.

Top tip: Spread the toes on the standing leg and press down, particularly into the big toe. This will help with balance.

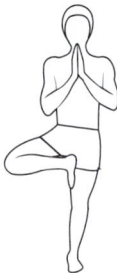

Corpse Pose (Shavasana/*Śavāsana*)

Come to rest on your back, legs stretched out, allowing your feet to fall open to the sides.

Bring your arms alongside your body, leaving some space between the body and arms. Palms facing upward, relax your hands and allow them to curl. Tuck your shoulder blades under, as if flattening the top of your back. Allow the outsides of your shoulders to relax down toward the ground. Lengthen the back of your neck and relax your whole body. Notice the places where the body meets the ground, allowing the body to sink into these spaces and feel completely supported.

Top tip: If resting flat on your mat is uncomfortable, try popping a pillow or a rolled-up mat underneath your knees.

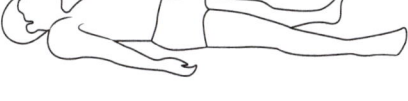

✦ VISUALIZATION: WHAT IS IT? ✦

Visualization meditation is a type of meditation that uses imagery instead of the breath to focus and hold attention. It's an immersive exercise that invites you to use all your senses, so it's not just what you see but also what you hear, smell, feel and even taste. Visualization can be so powerful that some studies have shown that the brain responds similarly to visualizing something as it does to actually doing it. This means that visualization meditation can help motivate you by making the brain believe the outcome is achievable.

It's not just about looking to the future, however. Visualization can also be a powerful way to create a sanctuary within yourself – a safe place you can return to at any time.

> **Top tip:** If you're having trouble focusing, try using a familiar location so your memory can help boost your visualization by providing reminders of what it feels like to be there.

✦ GETTING STARTED ✦

Visualization meditation can be self-directed or guided. There are a variety of techniques that can be used to practise visualization meditation, including:

- **Colour meditation:** This meditation involves turning whatever energy you want to cultivate more of in your life into a colour. For instance, you might imagine a calm blue. Each time you breathe in, you bring more of the colour into your body until eventually your whole body is full of the calm colour.

- **Creative visualization:** This technique is a powerful way to manifest desired goals and outcomes by using all the senses to imagine what it will be like when all your aspirations are achieved. Remember that your goals don't have to be material in nature; you can imagine things like what it would feel like to ace your presentation at work.

- **Peaceful place:** These meditations focus your mind's eye on a peaceful place. It could be somewhere you've been to, somewhere you aspire to go or somewhere wholly imagined.

EXERCISE: LOVING-KINDNESS MEDITATION

Loving-kindness meditation not only keeps us grounded in the present moment; it also fills that moment with love and compassion. It's a practice that cultivates positive emotions, and a desire for unconditional happiness for yourself and others. Follow these ten steps to spread loving-kindness to every being.

1 To begin, find a comfortable position that allows you to remain relaxed and alert. Settle into your breath.

2 Become aware of the breath in the region of the heart. Recall the feeling of being with someone you love. Someone who makes you feel happy. It could be a relative, partner, close friend or pet. Bring a picture of them into your mind and have a sense of them being next to you. Maybe you can feel some warmth spreading inside you. Perhaps you've started to smile. Keep feeling that love. Feel it flowing through your heart, maybe moving in rhythm with the breath. This is loving-kindness. It's a natural feeling that's accessible within us at any moment.

3 Keep a sense of your loved one in front of you and start to wish them well. Wish them the best. Wish them to be safe and protected, that they truly be happy.

4 Feel your loving-kindness growing stronger, flowing through your heart.

5 Allow the loving-kindness to grow; send it out to more people you know who are close to you. Wish them the best. Wish they be safe and protected, that they truly be happy.

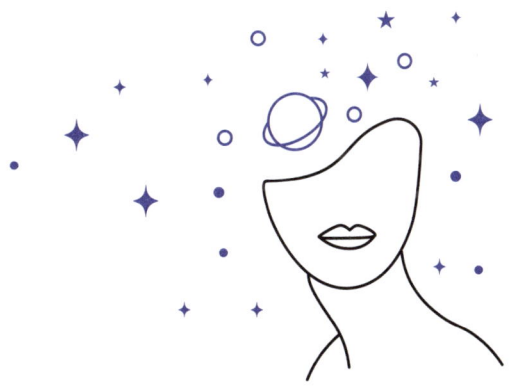

6 Imagine that your loved ones start to return the loving-kindness to you, wishing you are safe and protected, wishing you peace and true joy. See what arises in you as you feel this loving-kindness directed toward yourself. Ask yourself what you need to be happy, to be strong, to feel joy.

7 Keep a sense of that loving-kindness enveloping you and your loved ones and see if you can extend it even further. Send the loving-kindness out to people you know who are neutral to you and wish them the best. Wish them true joy and contentment.

8 Sense the loving-kindness like warmth or a light. Like a warm liquid with rippling waves, it spreads further, reaching even more people. Let it extend out to include the people you know whom you find challenging. Your loving-kindness has taken on an energy and strength of its own. It understands that many factors have influenced these problematic people and made them become a challenge for you. You wish that they be at peace. You wish that they be free from anxiety and worry.

9 As the loving-kindness spreads, it grows even stronger, reaching out to include even more people. Sense loving-kindness for everyone living in your country, whether you know them or not, whether you agree with them or not. May they be at peace. May they be free from anxiety and worry. May they feel joy.

10 Your loving-kindness is flowing in a rhythm, extending out now to all living beings on earth. Wish them all well. All types of animals, plants and people. May they all be healthy. May every living being be at ease. May we all experience joy. May we all be truly happy.

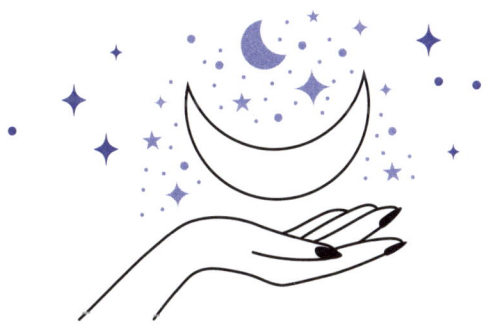

*To be fully alive, fully human,
and completely awake is to be
continually thrown out of the nest.*

PEMA CHÖDRÖN

✦ BREATH WORK: WHAT IS IT? ✦

Did you know that the average person breathes over 20,000 times daily? That's about 12 breaths each minute and about 7.5 million breaths a year. Considering our bodies perform an activity 20,000 times a day, it's incredible how little attention the breath is given. Breathing is an automatic process controlled by our nervous system, so lucky for us, the breath carries on even if we're not paying any attention at all.

Breath work is not just about becoming aware of the breath but also a mechanism for calming the body and mind. Paying attention to our breath can help us improve how we feel physically and how we interact with others. We can manipulate our breathing to achieve different outcomes. For instance, deep abdominal breathing will have a calming and grounding effect. Deep breathing can also improve our mood and increase our ability to focus. Imagine all that potential is available to you at no cost, 20,000 times a day, every single day. Powerful stuff!

✦ GETTING STARTED ✦

Start by checking in with your natural breathing patterns to see where the breath is at this moment in time. Does it feel shallow or deep? Are the inhales and the exhales the same length and the same strength? Is each breath the same length as the one before and the one to come, or is every third or fourth breath stronger than the others? Does each breath flow into the next like the waves of the ocean, or does the breath seem to get stuck?

You might want to make a mental note of any patterns you find through your breath observation. Do you notice your breath gets particularly shallow after stressful tasks? Do you breathe more easily when you sit down to eat your lunch or when having a conversation with a loved one? Understanding your current breathing patterns can show you where there might be room for improvement.

Once you spend a few moments observing your natural breath, you can start to engage in more mindful breathing by counting or noting the breath. This can be as simple as continuously repeating to yourself "breathing in, breathing out". Alternatively, you can count the length of the inhales and exhales, starting at one on the inhale to count its duration, and starting again at one on the exhale.

> **Top tip:** Try setting a timer to remind yourself to take breathing breaks throughout the day. Just a few minutes to close your eyes and focus on the breath can be beneficial.

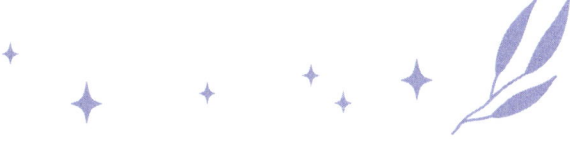

EXERCISE: FULL-BODY BREATHING

Full-body breathing helps root us in the present moment, fully aware of the body and the breath.

1 Close your eyes or soften your gaze, moving your focus inward. Become aware of your breath.

2 Inhale through the nose and feel the breath travelling down the left side of the body, all the way to your toes.

3 Exhale and feel the breath being pulled up the left side of the body, to the nose.

4 Inhale and feel the breath moving down the right side of your body.

5 Exhale and feel the breath travelling up the right side of the body, back to the nose, completing a full circle of breath around the body.

6 Feel this connection of the breath moving through the entire body, delivering oxygen and nutrients to all parts of your being.

Ask yourself: Where am I?
Answer: Here.
Ask yourself: What time is it?
Answer: Now.
Say it until you can hear it.

RAM DASS

DEVELOPING A MINDFULNESS PRACTICE

Now that you've seen how many ways there are to practise mindfulness, you're probably eager to get stuck in. Here are some helpful hints for developing your practice:

Be consistent

Making mindfulness a part of your everyday life is the best way to ensure it sticks. Pick a set time of day and stick to that commitment. Schedule it in your diary, put reminders on your phone and make it a priority. Keeping a mindfulness journal can help you to track your progress and keep you motivated.

Be realistic

Start small and build up over time. Mindfulness is not something to be mastered in months or possibly even years. It's a continuous practice that will evolve over your lifetime. Just as the circumstances of your life will change, your practice will grow and adapt.

Be patient

Practise with patience; it won't be a straight line to success. There will be good days and not-so-good days. The trick is not to get too attached to either outcome. While it's nice to acknowledge successes, it's just as important to recognize inevitable setbacks. Developing your mindfulness muscles will take time.

Be persistent

Overcoming obstacles is an important part of your mindfulness development. There will always be reasons not to practise. Making mindfulness a priority will help you stay on track and stick to your schedule. Remembering the benefits of mindfulness will help keep you motivated.

Be flexible

Life happens. Sometimes, even the best-laid plans get knocked out of play. We can allow for some flexibility in our mindfulness practice. Can't get to yoga? Then perhaps you fit in a body scan before bedtime. With so many ways to practise mindfulness, there's always something we can do to stay dedicated to our practice.

✦ CREATING THE RIGHT ✦ ENVIRONMENT

Though mindfulness can be practised almost anytime and anywhere, some environments can enhance our practice, and some will challenge it. A space that feels comfortable and inviting acts as an incentive if we're procrastinating. If we're lucky enough to create these peaceful places, they can become part of our visualization practice, as our sanctuary from chaos.

You don't need a large physical location for setting up your sanctuary. In fact, smaller spaces can feel cosier and hold the energy more closely, but there are a few things to consider when creating your space:

- **Air:** Where possible, fresh air is ideal in your mindfulness space.

- **Cleanliness:** You'll want your space to be free from dust and clutter. A clear and open space is most conducive to mindfulness.

- **Comfort:** Make your mindfulness space a place of comfort. To make it inviting, you can use cushions and bolsters, blankets or wraps. Add plants for an additional boost from nature.

- **Disruptions:** Can you close the door to your mindfulness space, or is it somewhere that others know not to disturb you?

- **Lighting:** Low lighting or even candlelight is much more inviting than harsh overhead lighting. Fairy lights or battery-operated candles also work well.

- **Noise:** Is there a lot of external noise audible from your mindfulness space? It's not always possible to find silent spaces in our busy lives, but we should avoid areas with loud or constant background noise when possible.

- **Scent:** Where possible, choose an area that is not exposed to powerful smells. You might want to add a scent of your choice through incense, candles or an essential oil diffuser.

- **Temperature:** If it's too hot or cold, you'll have trouble sitting still for very long. Also, try to avoid draughty spaces.

✦ MINDFULNESS COMMUNITIES ✦

Mindfulness doesn't have to be a solo adventure. In fact, being part of a mindfulness community can help you through the inevitable rough patches. Having others to encourage you when you're struggling or cheer you on when you're making progress can make your mindfulness journey more enjoyable. There's comfort in knowing that others have been where you are now.

Finding a mindfulness community is probably easier than you think. Many mindfulness instructors organize gatherings, including social elements, to draw the community together. Alternatively, you can join online mindfulness communities. These can be found on social media sites and websites that list events. Some of these communities are global, with thousands of members worldwide, and some might be more localized to your area.

If you're feeling inspired, look for mindfulness retreats. Many teachers organize weekend or week-long retreats in different locations. Some will incorporate different forms of mindfulness, like a yoga and meditation retreat, while others might be day-long workshops with the opportunity to practise in a group setting.

The only way to live is by accepting each minute as an unrepeatable miracle.

STORM JAMESON

✦ POTENTIAL CHALLENGES ✦

Even the most dedicated practitioners will face obstacles along the way. While creating new habits, it's common to stumble and fall back on old patterns of thought and behaviour. We're often so goal-driven and programmed to expect results that learning to simply be where we are without judgement is a mental shift that takes time. Common roadblocks include:

- **Distraction:** We've moved away from human beings to human doings – we're so used to being in motion that slowing down is bound to be met with resistance.

- **Doubt:** Mindfulness may not be noticeable to you or the outside world. We don't win medals for mindfulness, and no one will compliment you on your new mindful outlook. Without markers of our progress, it's easy to get discouraged and begin to doubt our abilities.

- **Pain:** Though mindfulness can help us manage our pain response, there are times when pain can overwhelm our ability to act mindfully. When this happens, we first need to manage the pain as best we can and then we can return to our mindfulness ways.

- **Stress:** When your body is having a physiological response to stress, it can be in "fight or flight" mode. At times like this, mindfulness can feel unreachable.

- **Time:** With 101 things on your to-do list, finding time for slowing down can feel like an impractical luxury.

- **Tiredness/hunger:** Feelings of tiredness or hunger can throw us out of kilter and override our attempts at mindfulness. Addressing these basic needs before any formal practice will minimize distractions.

Recognizing these forms of resistance for what they are – biological, situational or fear-based reactions – will take some of the energy from them and we can celebrate that acceptance as a sign of progress.

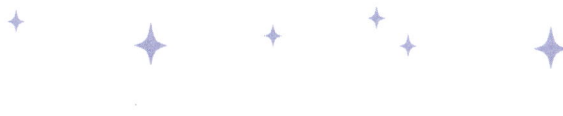

✦ BEGINNER'S MINDSET ✦

Everything feels exciting when we're learning something new. As we gain experience and exposure, sometimes we lose our open-mindedness and enthusiasm. Keeping that beginner's mindset alive, even within our most routine activities, can enhance our thinking and help us to continue learning.

The beginner's mindset concept comes from Zen Buddhism. Known as *shoshin*, it's the idea of approaching everything you see as if for the first time. It encourages an attitude of openness and curiosity in whatever you do, whether for the first or fortieth time.

Being open to new possibilities allows for different outcomes; we stop letting the past dictate our future. A beginner's mindset encourages asking questions and exploring options, so rather than feeling stuck in endless repetition, new ideas and approaches are considered. This mindset doesn't mean disregarding any of your relevant skills or knowledge – you can use them while remaining curious and open to new ideas.

Why adopt a beginner's mindset?

A beginner's mindset transforms your thinking, learning and even your interactions with others. By not engaging in rigid thinking, you allow for endless possibilities. Just because something occurred in the past doesn't mean it's destined to happen in the future. A beginner's mindset can contribute to:

- **Better problem-solving skills:** A beginner's mindset turns challenges into opportunities, meaning you explore strategies and solutions with positivity and an open mind.

- **Enhanced innovation and creativity:** Letting go of preconceived thinking unlocks creativity. Fresh perspectives encourage new ideas, rather than falling back on what has always been done before.

- **Increased resilience:** The ability to be flexible, adjusting your ideas and expectations, makes you more resilient when things don't go to plan.

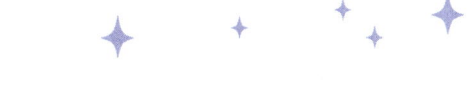

CHAPTER THREE

EVERYDAY
MINDFULNESS

Once you've learned the basics, you'll find that integrating mindfulness into everyday life can bring feelings of immense calm and clarity. This chapter explores practical ways to embrace mindfulness in daily activities like walking, eating, doing chores, conversations or while engaging in screen time. You'll find tips and exercises for enhancing your daily life with moments of stillness and connection. Whether it's at work, at home or in quiet moments alone, mindfulness enhances our connection to the present moment and deepens our relationships. By embracing gratitude, patience and presence, you'll find balance and joy amidst the busyness of life.

EVERYDAY RITUALS TO LIVE MORE MINDFULLY

Rituals can transform ordinary activities into more meaningful events. Instead of moving through our day on autopilot, we operate with awareness and presence. They can also infuse meaning into what might otherwise feel mundane, reframing ordinary activities as enjoyable and even turning them into something we anticipate. Here are some ways to cultivate mindful rituals:

Morning meditation

Our first few moments after awakening are impressionable and can set the tone for the day ahead. Before reaching for your phone and letting outside influences in, try spending a few moments in quiet meditation.

Intention setting

Setting an intention in the morning for the day ahead can help you choose your actions more mindfully. For example, you can set an intention to embrace your full range of emotions or to seek joy in your surroundings. Check in at specific points in the day to see how well you are adhering to your intention.

Natural connection

Make time in your day to immerse yourself in nature. Even in the busiest cities, green and blue spaces exist for connecting with the natural world. If you only have a small patch of grass to work with, take your shoes off and feel the earth under your feet.

An attitude of gratitude

End your day by spending a few moments listing three things you are grateful for – it could be things that happened in the day or constants that sustain you routinely.

Reflect and reset

Journalling is a great mindfulness practice that allows time for reflection and is a way to let go of unexpressed feelings. Writing them down can release their energy while also providing perspective. Sometimes, seeing things in black and white makes them feel much more manageable.

✦ EATING MINDFULLY ✦

Mindful eating, a mindfulness practice originating from Buddhism, can help enhance your appreciation of food, encourage better food choices and even improve your gut health. Here are seven steps to eat more mindfully:

1 **Tune in to what your body is telling you:** Mindful eating happens when we're hungry, not when the clock tells us it's time to eat or to fill an emotional hole. Wait for your body to feel hungry, instead of your mind saying it's time to eat.

2 **Take a seat:** Try to avoid eating on the go. Take time away from your busy routine to enjoy your meal.

3 **Recognize the food chain:** Before your first bite, take a moment to recognize all the work that went into the meal before you. Considering both its preparation and the individual ingredients, how many people played a part in making the meal you're about to enjoy? Offer appreciation for

the abundance of effort that goes into delivering your meal.

4   **Engage all your senses:** Notice the range of colours on your plate. Inhale any aromas. Taste for texture, temperature and flavour.

5   **Think small:** Eat with a smaller plate or bowl to limit your portion size. Take small bites and chew each one thoroughly. You may be surprised by how much flavour comes from food that is savoured slowly.

6   **Slow down:** There's no prize for finishing first in eating. Take your time and eat slowly. Put your fork down in-between bites. Try not to multi-task while eating. Other than engaging in conversation with others, leave your to-do list for later. Mindful eating can also be practised alone and in silence.

7   **Press pause:** Take a few minutes of rest after eating rather than running off to your next activity. Linger for a while, allowing time for digestion.

✦ MINDFUL COMMUNICATION ✦

Bringing aspects of mindfulness to our communication with others can have a profound effect on our relationships. Mindful listening can make you a much more effective and empathetic communicator. When you give your full attention to the person speaking, seeking to understand not just what they are saying but the intention and emotion behind it, you take your interactions to a deeper level. Making others feel heard and understood makes them feel respected and valued, which can soften even the most challenging relationships.

Benefits
Mastering the art of mindful listening has many personal and professional benefits including:

- **Clarity of thinking:** Thorough listening allows for a more objective assessment of situations without making assumptions or jumping to conclusions.

- **Deepening relationships:** Good communication is the foundation for strong connections. When people feel heard they are more likely to open up and share their true selves.

- **Improved awareness:** Mindful listening can help us understand more about our triggers, feelings and reactions as we notice what arises in our thoughts.

- **Minimizing conflict:** Thoughtful listening can reduce disagreements. Where differences of opinion remain, they can often be mutually respected.

- **Understanding the full picture:** Mindful listening includes paying attention to non-verbal cues, which often fill in the blanks of what isn't being communicated in words.

Top tip: Remember the difference between reacting and responding when it's your time to speak. Reacting is usually a quick, emotionally driven response. Responding is a thoughtful and measured reply that considers potential outcomes and chooses an emotionally intelligent option that aligns with the speaker's values. When in doubt, pause for a deep breath before replying!

✦ HOW TO LISTEN ✦ MORE MINDFULLY

Like other aspects of mindfulness, learning to listen mindfully takes time. It's likely to present challenges at first as you work to create new listening habits.

Pay attention fully

Listening requires full attention. Focus your attention entirely on the person speaking and what's being said. Eye contact shows the speaker that you're engaged in listening. Checking your phone shows them that you are not.

Avoid interrupting

It might be tempting to intervene at certain times, particularly if it's a subject you feel strongly about, but this is just the time to stay quiet.

Stay focused

Train your mind not to wander. When you notice it happening, gently draw your focus back to the conversation.

Look between the lines

Some studies rank nonverbal communication as more expressive than spoken words! Think of all you'd miss if looking elsewhere when someone is talking to you.

Ask for clarification

If there's anything you're uncertain about, don't be afraid to ask the speaker to clarify their meaning.

Summarize your understanding

Repeating back your understanding of what's been said will help the speaker clarify or confirm that what you've heard is what they intended.

Mindful listening shows that you value the other person's input and respect their opinion. It allows time for consideration before responding and can diffuse tension from a situation. Honing your mindful listening skills can improve relationships with colleagues, friends and loved ones.

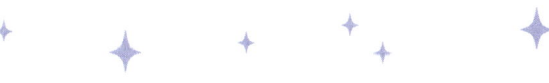

MINDFULNESS IN HOUSEHOLD CHORES

You don't have to be religious to appreciate the meaning of the well-known phrase "God is in the details". There is something therapeutic about the process (and result!) of cleaning and tidying. Not only that, applying mindfulness to tasks like washing the dishes has been linked to lowering stress and boosting creativity. In fact, mundane tasks can soothe mental chatter as the mind rests in the rhythm of repetition. Plus, there's the bonus of a pleasant result at the end.

Tidying up

Disorganization can make it hard to relax and reduce productivity. Clutter can also be a sign of a lack of clarity in other areas of life, including mentally. A well-organized space fosters a feeling of calm and spaciousness.

Washing dishes

While washing dishes, take time to notice the temperature of the water, the scent of the washing-up liquid and the simple yet symbolic pleasure of wiping a plate clean.

Sweeping

Like washing up, the repetitive nature of sweeping and mopping symbolizes creating a clean slate. As you sweep up physical dust, imagine you are equally clearing the corners of your mind.

Laundry

Folding laundry is one of life's simple pleasures. Notice the smell of freshly cleaned clothes and the different colours and textures of the fabrics. Turning a messy pile of clothes into well-folded, neat stacks is an excellent opportunity to help untangle thoughts.

Top tip: Be particular about the cleaning products you use, especially if they are strongly scented. When you're finished cleaning, why not light a scented candle to further enhance the atmosphere?

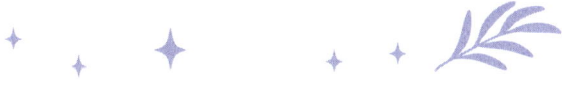

✦ MONEY MINDFULNESS ✦

Managing finances can be a source of great stress. Applying the principles of mindfulness to your spending habits can transform your relationship with money. Mindful spending cuts down on emotional or impulse purchases, which might feel good in the moment but aren't aligned with your financial goals.

Smart spending requires thought and discipline – two characteristics cultivated through mindfulness. Being more in control of your finances can lower stress and lead to greater overall well-being. Here are some tips to help you become more mindful of money:

- **Create:** Develop a conscious budget that allocates enough for your necessities, including an amount for enjoyment when possible. A mindful spending plan needs a long-term outlook, not a short-term squeeze.

- **Pause:** Before you make any purchases, consider whether they align with your financial goals. If you're unsure, delay the decision to buy for a bit longer.

- **Plan:** Developing a long-term financial plan can help you to be mindful of your everyday spending. It's much easier to skip the daily coffee habit when you know that money is going toward your upcoming holiday.

- **Purchase:** When you do make a purchase, try to pay in cash. Sometimes, the simple act of seeing how much something costs will either make you reconsider or make you appreciate more whatever you are acquiring.

- **Track:** Start keeping tabs on all your incoming funds and outgoing expenses. Seeing the sums in black and white can sometimes lead to surprising discoveries.

Engaging in mindfulness techniques when considering what you're buying and why can transform your spending habits. Mindful money management will help you stick to your budget, save money and reduce stress.

Be present, be patient, be gentle, be kind... everything else will take care of itself.

ANDY PUDDICOMBE, QUOTING A FORMER TEACHER

✦ MINDFULNESS AT WORK ✦

Work environments can be a leading cause of stress in our lives. Deadlines, meetings, targets, colleagues and clients can all contribute to workplace challenges. Mindfulness in the workplace can not only make us better at our jobs but also more motivated to do them. It might not magically write your reports for you, but it can bring a range of benefits including:

- Better decision-making
- Enhanced creativity and innovation
- Greater overall job satisfaction
- Improved relationships with colleagues
- More focus and productivity
- Reduced stress and burnout

Incorporating mindfulness principles like "responding – not reacting" will help to foster smoother relationships with colleagues, while approaching problems with a beginner's mindset will encourage creativity.

HOW TO BE MORE MINDFUL AT WORK

Set a schedule
Plan out your schedule in advance. Break large projects down into shorter deliverables and use daily/weekly action plans to stay focused on the task at hand rather than running through mental to-do lists.

Cultivate calm
Create a calm workspace by tidying your desk, bringing some of the outside world in with plants and playing soothing music (or even white noise) to drown out external distractions.

Take breaks
Short breaks can help you stay focused. Taking a few minutes to walk, stretch and breathe will do wonders for your ability to concentrate.

Stay hydrated
Caffeine might seem like a good idea at the time, but drinking water is a better option for staying focused.

Turn off notifications

Set times to check your emails rather than scanning them throughout the day. Silence non-essential notifications.

Communicate mindfully

Think before you reply, ask clarifying questions of colleagues and consider your own choice of words when explaining your position. When dealing with difficult colleagues, first try to find common ground before expressing any disagreement.

Monotask

Studies have shown that although it might make you feel more productive, multi-tasking leads to decreased productivity. Instead, focus on one activity or action point, take it to its conclusion or stopping point and move on to the next action. You'll find it quicker to get through tasks, and there's less risk of error.

Practise gratitude

Say thank you to colleagues when they are helpful. Thank people publicly when appropriate. Recognize achievements within your team and with clients.

✦ MINDFUL LEADERSHIP ✦

Creating a culture of mindfulness in the workplace starts at the top. Leaders can set the tone for developing a compassionate culture that encourages communication and creativity. Mindful leaders are meticulous in their communication and understand that their actions have a ripple effect through their teams. Far from the authoritative management of old, mindful leadership is collaborative and won't focus solely on an end goal or result – but it will recognize its impact on staff in achieving it.

Mindful leadership can have a marked impact on staff morale, motivation and, ultimately, the success of the business. Mindful leaders share similar qualities, including:

- **Attention:** Practising mindful listening to comprehend without judgement.

- **Authenticity:** Admitting individual shortcomings or failures and sharing successes among the team.

- **Balance:** Weighing up organizational goals in tandem with team impact.

- **Compassion:** Showing genuine concern for the well-being of the team.

- **Creativity:** Maintaining a beginner's mindset to encourage creativity and innovation in themselves and their team.

- **Decisiveness:** Gathering necessary information before making a decision. Ensuring decisions align with team values and goals.

- **Patience:** Exhibiting patience and allowing team members the time they need to learn, grow and excel.

- **Reflection:** Accepting feedback from all directions without fear.

Mindful leaders can pave the way to higher satisfaction levels within the workplace, showcasing the positive impacts of mindfulness in action.

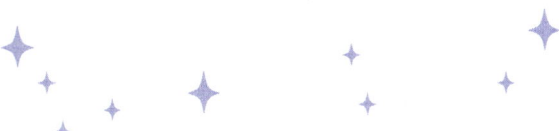

MINDFULNESS IN RELATIONSHIPS

Positive relationships, enhanced by mindfulness, are a great motivator and not only make us happier, but can also make us healthier. Strong social connections are a leading indicator of our longevity. Plus, it's not about the number of close relationships we have; it's about nurturing the quality of the ones we do. Utilizing mindfulness techniques can help strengthen already strong relationships and even smooth over challenging ones.

Stronger relationships through mindfulness

Building and nurturing relationships is one of the best investments we can make with our time. Here are some simple ways to get started:

- **Find common ground:** Nurturing connection is about finding commonalities. This could be common backgrounds, beliefs or shared experiences. We could share a sense of humour or particular interests. We build stronger bonds when we focus on what we have in common rather than our differences.

- **Kindness is key:** It sounds so simple, but kindness is key to strong relationships. When we take time to mindfully respond instead of reacting, we can treat others with more respect and kindness. It's much easier to show vulnerability to someone who is kind, diffusing anger and eliminating embarrassment. Likewise, being kind to others makes us feel better about ourselves.

- **Live and let go:** Sometimes there are relationships that just aren't good for us. This could be for a variety of reasons, but the end result is that they end up taking more away from us than they give. When we recognize this, we need to minimize our exposure where possible.

SIX MINDFUL RELATIONSHIP HABITS

Here are some mindfulness-based relationship habits that will ensure the needs of both you and your partner are met:

1 **Pay attention:** Be fully present when having conversations. Put phones away and turn off televisions or other distractions.

2 **Listen fully:** Practise mindful listening – hear what is being said without judgement and without jumping ahead to formulate a response.

3 **Express gratitude:** Tell your partner when they've done something you appreciate.

4 **Respond, don't react:** In times of stress, pause, breathe and respond rationally to challenges, framing them as something that you face together.

5 **Mind the little things:** Pay attention to the small details – ask your partner what makes them feel good and try to repeat these actions often.

6 **Be intentional:** Develop goals as a couple, creating a shared vision.

Forever –
is composed of Nows.

EMILY DICKINSON

MINDFULNESS AND TECHNOLOGY

The phrase "digital detox" has become as much a part of our language as tech itself. Whether you're old enough to remember life before mobile phones or a digital native who grew up with a small screen, technology is a firm fixture in everyday life. Our handheld devices act not just as a means of communication but as libraries, maps, dictionaries and radios. We're so reliant on them that we sometimes forget that we need time away from our small screens to remember the bigger picture. Mindfulness reminds us to be present in our surroundings, not in a digital dreamworld.

There are many reasons why a regular digital detox is a good idea. Though tech can make our lives easier and improve productivity, it can also be a source of great stress. Being connected all the time or feeling the constant need to check notifications and messages can lead to increased anxiety. Mindfulness techniques can help us develop a more balanced approach to our tech use and reduce the impact of our digital interactions.

A digital detox might be right for you if:

- You check for messages or notifications every few minutes.

- You feel anxious if you don't know where your phone is at all times.

- You feel compelled to monitor the likes and comments on your social media posts.

- You feel jealous, angry or stressed after viewing social media sites.

- You need to check your phone before you can concentrate on other things.

Using planned breaks from tech is a great way to reduce your exposure and reliance on it without forgoing all the benefits it can bring.

MINDFUL VERSUS MINDLESS TECH TIME

Time away from tech can benefit your well-being and reset your digital relationship. A detox is an opportunity to set boundaries around mindful use of tech, rather than mindlessly doomscrolling.

When you're ready, choose a combination of mindfulness techniques to reduce your screen time by swapping mindless habits for mindful ones:

Mindless: Allowing all push notifications.
Mindful: Allowing only essential notifications.

Mindless: Keeping your tech devices with you at all times.
Mindful: Planning tech-free times around meals and having an evening cut-off time, spending time outdoors with your phone for emergency use only and using tech at preplanned times.

Mindless: Scrolling before bed.
Mindful: Keeping tech devices out of the bedroom entirely.

Mindless: Connecting with and following hundreds of people.
Mindful: Keeping your connections to close friends, family and content with values that align with your own.

Mindless: Overusing social media apps.
Mindful: Using apps that track your time online and limit your screen time.

Mindless: Engaging with friends and family only through social media and messaging.
Mindful: Making plans to meet in person to spend time with your loved ones.

Mindless: Scrolling endlessly through random websites.
Mindful: Purposely engaging with uplifting content.

Awareness is the first step toward creating a more balanced approach to your relationship with technology. Mindfulness teaches us that each moment is precious. Before picking up your device ask yourself if what you're about to do is purposeful and will bring joy or connection. If it doesn't meet those criteria, consider whether it's necessary.

✦ MINDFUL BY NATURE ✦

The natural world can invoke feelings of wonder and a sense of awe at the beauty of Mother Nature. We feel grounded and at peace when we're connected to the earth. It reminds us to tread more lightly on our natural home and often releases our endless need to excel and achieve. Being immersed in nature, we're aware of the cycle of life, the rhythm of the seasons and may feel all of our senses are engaged.

Immersing ourselves in nature helps improve our physical and mental health. Doctors in Scotland have started prescribing time in nature to specific patient groups. Studies have shown that people who are more connected with nature are usually happier overall, as nature can promote calmness, creativity and joy. It can also improve our attention and lower stress, similar to mindfulness practices. Combining the two – practising mindfulness while immersed in nature – is a powerful and deeply satisfying experience.

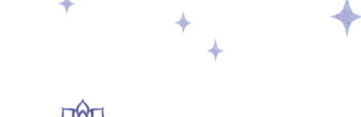

Nature connectedness

Nature connectedness is a scientifically accepted term describing our connection to the natural world. Studies on green and blue spaces, even in busy urban environments, show how powerful short bursts of time in the natural world can be – being surrounded by a forest of trees can help to slow down one's heart rate and soften facial muscles. Just 15 minutes of exposure can reduce cortisol levels (a hormone strongly linked to stress). Spending time in nature can increase alpha waves in the brain, sending calming signals to the body.

Practising mindfulness in the natural world can enhance our mindful time and connection to nature. Getting outside might also be a more accessible path to mindfulness for those who prefer more active relaxation.

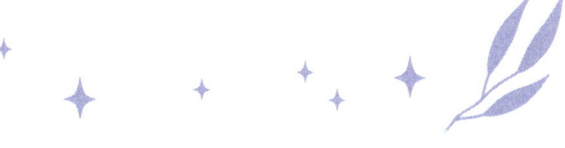

NOTICING NATURE: GOING OUTSIDE TO GO INSIDE

You don't need to find a forest in the middle of nowhere to engage with nature. It's possible to foster a natural connection in small green spaces or even by stargazing or listening to birdsong.

Observe

How many other living beings can you see as you sit or walk in a natural environment? Not just animals but also plants, trees, mosses, birds and bugs. Take time to note all the life around you on the ground, in the air and even in the water.

Move

Move mindfully, connecting to each motion. Notice the ground beneath you, its texture and terrain. Hear any sounds you create from treading on earth. Listen for other sounds around you.

Pause

Find a peaceful place and pause. Engage all of your senses as you tune in to what surrounds you. Focus your attention on something small – a single flower or leaf on a tree. Note the finer detail of it. Move back and marvel at how many flowers and leaves there are in your more expansive view.

Go with the flow
Find some water to engage with – even a small pond or rain falling. What sounds can you hear? Does the rain have a smell? Being near water has been scientifically proven to improve our well-being.

Connect
Try to observe any energies and processes that are happening around you. Can you see animals feeding their young? Where is there movement, and where is there stillness? Where is new life or growth occurring? Engage with the entire life cycle of nature.

Journal
Take a notebook outdoors and write how you feel when immersed in nature. Do you notice any difference in your breathing or mood? Perhaps engage in free writing, simply writing down any words that come into your consciousness.

SUSTAINING A MINDFUL LIFESTYLE

Embarking on a mindfulness journey can feel exciting. There's so much to learn, and you'll likely feel encouraged to continue once you start experiencing the benefits. As time goes on, there will be challenges to stay on track with your mindfulness practices. Remember that progress is not a straight line. There are often pitfalls on the path to success. Mindfulness is a way of life; it's not a goal to achieve. There will always be more to learn and ways to improve.

Similarly, mindfulness doesn't disappear at the flick of a switch. When we lose our temper, find ourselves giving in to strong emotions or skipping our meditation sessions, we don't lose all our mindfulness and start again from scratch.

The key to staying motivated is to start slowly and be realistic about goals. It might be that practising five minutes of mindfulness a day is all we can achieve for the first 30 days. That's still an impressive 150 minutes of mindfulness – an excellent foundation for growth.

Find practices that work for you and fit into your lifestyle. If the only yoga studio is over 30 minutes from your home or work, how much will you realistically go? Are there other options, like online classes, that you can do from home?

Remember you can incorporate small acts of mindfulness throughout your day – for example, mindful walking or starting each day with a clear intention, like, "I will pause before speaking today."

Once you find practices you enjoy and that fit in your schedule, you'll look forward to them rather than feel like they're an imposition.

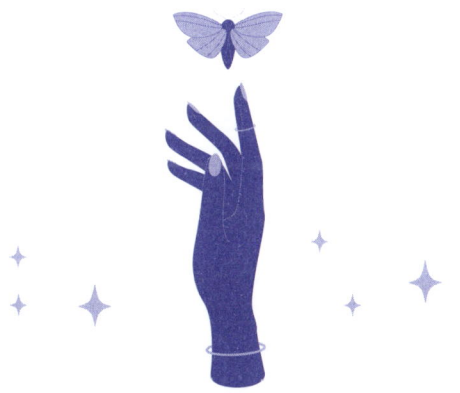

✦ EASY EVERYDAY MINDFULNESS ✦

Even with the best-laid plans, sometimes life happens, and we need to change and adapt. Mindfulness teaches us resilience for times like these. Remember, mindfulness can be brought into your life every day in small but significant ways, for example:

- **Brushing teeth:** Notice the taste, texture and smell of your toothpaste.

- **Commuting:** Notice the people or cars around you. Become aware of any emotions arising in you, particularly when delays occur.

- **Journalling:** Make a habit of keeping a gratitude list, starting or ending each day with three things you're grateful for.

- **Washing hands:** What does the water feel like when it touches your skin. Is it hot? Cold?

Finally, seek out positive people to build your support system. When you surround yourself with others who share your interests it makes the journey even more enjoyable!

Breathing in, I calm my body
and mind. Breathing out, I smile.
Dwelling in the present moment,
I know this is the only moment.

THÍCH NHẤT HẠNH

✦ CONCLUSION ✦

Modern mindfulness has expanded beyond its religious roots to encompass broader applications in mental well-being, stress reduction and personal growth. This book highlights why it's important to honour the traditional aspects of mindfulness while still embracing its evolution into a method for navigating the complexities of modern life. The full impact of all the positive ways mindfulness can boost well-being is still unknown, but it's important to remember that it's not a cure-all solution.

One of the most exciting aspects of mindfulness is its versatility. It can be practised many ways in a variety of settings. Mindfulness needs no equipment or special clothing. It doesn't require a huge time commitment or cost anything. You can be mindful at home, at work and even while commuting between the two.

Bringing mindfulness into your life can help you manage stress, enhance your emotional resilience and cultivate deeper connections with yourself and your loved ones. Integrating mindfulness into your daily routine will not only enrich your life – it can create a ripple effect of positivity that inspires those around you. Embrace the journey and remember that every moment of mindfulness is a step toward a more balanced, joyful life.

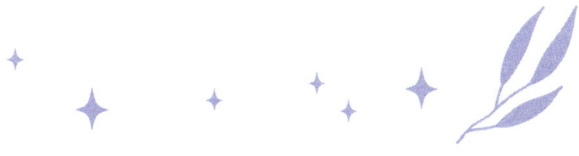

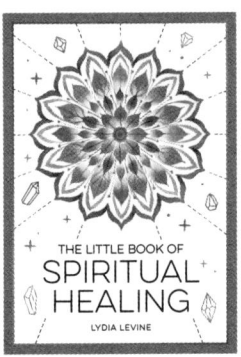

**THE LITTLE BOOK OF
SPIRITUAL HEALING**
Lydia Levine

Paperback 978-1-83799-366-6

Restore and rejuvenate your mind, body and soul with this modern introduction to the ancient wisdom of energy therapies. From Ayurveda and acupuncture to crystals and chakra healing, this treasury of information holds everything you need to know about holistic healing methods in order to embark on your own personal journey to health and harmony.

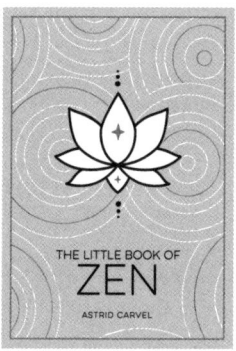

THE LITTLE BOOK OF ZEN
Astrid Carvel

Paperback 978-1-80007-197-1

Zen is a philosophy for living in a state of kindness, gratitude and awareness, teaching us to be present and to experience the world as it truly is. This book will guide you through the concept of Zen, revealing how you can apply its principles to your daily life and how you can reap the benefits to gain a greater sense of peace and calm.

Have you enjoyed this book? If so, find us on
Facebook at **Summersdale Publishers**, on
Twitter/X at **@Summersdale** and on Instagram and
TikTok at **@summersdalebooks** and get in touch.

We'd love to hear from you!

www.summersdale.com